Rosa Ruoppo

The Application of Artificial Intelligence in Alzheimer's Disease

Rosa Ruoppo

The Application of Artificial Intelligence in Alzheimer's Disease

A modern approach of technology applied to medicine to counter the evolution of Alzheimer's disease

ScienciaScripts

INTRODUCTION

In this text we enunciate how, through the use of technology, mainly Artificial Intelligence, we can deepen the study of a disease with a widespread epidemiological picture and whose causes are not yet well known: Alzheimer's disease. It is crucial to focus on research for the study of this disease since, among the many symptoms detected, it involves memory deficits leading the patient to total isolation.

Current focus is on technological progress and its impact in today's society, especially in health care.

Through extensive research and multiple studies, it is predicted that the combination of technological innovation with medicine could be a turning point for the study, prevention and diagnosis of many diseases including dementia.

In pursuing this goal, there is a tendency to describe Alzheimer's disease in its entirety by evaluating the different phases of the patient's care management as a whole, moving from the use of obsolete pharmacological and psychosocial treatments and diagnosis to a reality focused on the use of new technological methods; therefore, a model of robotics will be under development that can provide care for the elderly with dementia, helping them not only to have an approach with technology, but they will be able to use it in order to care for themselves, so through artificial intelligence there is a tendency not only to improve and refine knowledge of the disease itself, but the Health System will be able to make use of it to offer excellent services to patients, as a result there will be a health care based on a model 4.0

1. ALZHEIMER'S DISEASE: A GLOBAL VIEW OF THE DISEASE

1.1 Discovery and description of dementia

The term dementia comes from the Latin word 'demens' meaning 'to be out of one's mind.' This word was first coined in the 13th century, but in the medical world it was not recognized until the 18th century. Initially by the Greeks it was regarded as a very specific neurodegenerative disease that concerned only human senility and its degeneration related to a main disease-Alzheimer's disease-but in reality it encompassed every psychiatric and neurological condition leading to psychosocial consequences. Later with the discovery of other forms related to it, but especially to old age, it took on a broader meaning, changing to indicate a group of neurodegenerative diseases of the brain typical of old age and characterized by an irreversible and gradual reduction of cognitive faculties, such as memory loss, which is part of the so-called "Memory Disorders," such that it interferes with daily life. Those suffering from such disorders were referred to special specialists called "alienists."

Sometimes there is a tendency to associate dementia with so-called "cognitive decline," but although they result in very similar manifestations, in fact doctors tend to point out that they are two different conditions, in fact, such cognitive impairment, being typical of old age, is a normal involutional process that the brain undergoes, during aging, this involves a gradual reduction in brain volume, the loss of several neurons and inefficient transmission of nerve signals. However, in some cases, this condition can cause mild cognitive impairment, leading to overt memory deficits or more severe forms of dementia. Mild cognitive impairment is thus a clinical finding somewhere between natural human aging and the onset of dementia: it often does not impair the normal functions or quality of life of the affected person, as only small areas of the brain are deteriorated that do not completely change the neurological complex. However, it does affect the ability to perform complex tasks and can predict worsening of the condition to dementia or Alzheimer's disease.

Alzheimer's disease was first described in 1906 by German psychiatrist and neuropathologist Alois Alzheimer. The patient first diagnosed with Alzheimer's disease was a 51-year-old woman, Auguste Deter, who presented with various symptoms, including short-term memory loss, associated with sudden mood changes. After the woman's death, Alzheimer obtained her medical records and examined the brain in detail with the help of other physicians, including the Italian Gaetano Perusini, and found that the encephalon exhibited histological features other than normal i.e. massive neuronal loss and the presence of amyloid plaques and neurofibrillary tangles. After studying several other cases, Alzheimer presented his findings at the Tübingen Psychiatric Conference in 1907, but his beliefs were initially met with skepticism. Slowly, the theory began to spread, arriving in the year 1910, when Emil Kraepelin, one of the founders of modern psychiatry, republished his "Treatise on Psychiatry"-which became the real centerpiece of the field-in which he defined Alzheimer's disease as a real disease.

Alzheimer's disease is a neurodegenerative disease that involves a gradual and irreversible loss of cognitive function; it is a form of dementia that appears in old age but can also affect young people between 30 and 60 years old, also called early Alzheimer's or juvenile Alzheimer's.

This disease is known to cause memory lapses, speech problems, personality changes, lack of initiative, confusion, disorientation, loss of thinking and judgment. Alzheimer's disease reduces a patient's life expectancy in fact, advanced complications of the disease can even lead to death.

1.2 Morphology, pathogenesis and biochemistry

Studies by MRI and PET scan on the brains of patients with Alzheimer's disease have shown that there are significant abnormalities in the brain organ. The following are the most important ones:

- Cerebral Atrophy in Alzheimer's Disease

First, the process of brain atrophy appears in the cerebral cortex and some cortical areas.

Brain atrophy refers to a decrease in brain tissue volume due to necrosis or shrinkage of neurons.

Especially in patients with Alzheimer's disease, brain atrophy from the onset of the disease mainly affects the medial part of the temporal lobe, where the hippocampus, amygdala, entorhinal cortex, and parahippocampal cortex are located; several studies confirm that this evidence is consistent with the clinical features of Alzheimer's disease, particularly memory loss: the aforementioned brain regions, in fact, control memories and short- and long-term storage processes.

In the case of medial temporal lobe atrophy in Alzheimer's disease, it is certainly worth mentioning that this is a phenomenon that is evident from the onset of the first symptoms and is bound to worsen until the later stages of the disease.

There are studies that have compared brain changes caused by Alzheimer's disease and normal aging i.e., cognitive decline. In contrast to Alzheimer's disease, age-related cognitive decline is associated with small volume changes affecting regions of the prefrontal cortex, insular cortex, anterior cingulate lobe, superior temporal lobe, inferior parietal lobe, and precuneus (superior parietal lobe); although it does not seem to affect the hippocampus and the brain regions most closely related to it since no volume changes in gray matter are noted.

However, it is also important to note that the atrophic process caused by Alzheimer's disease is not limited to the medial temporal lobe; in fact, several studies have shown that it also affects the medial parietal lobe from the beginning and during the duration of the disease, and only in the moderately advanced stages of the disease the frontal lobe and brainstem (especially the midbrain).

-    Dilation of Cerebral Ventricles in Alzheimer's Disease

In patients with Alzheimer's disease, another important abnormality observed in the brain is dilation of the lateral ventricles and sometimes the third ventricle.

The increase in ventricular volume observed in Alzheimer's patients is secondary to the process of brain atrophy: ventricular cavities gradually increase as brain tissue shrinks.

Pathogenesis

Microscopic studies show that brain atrophy results from the formation of protein aggregates that have a toxic effect on neurons and synapses in the brain.

In fact, the brains of Alzheimer's patients have heavy clusters of proteins, both extracellular and intracellular, that are not present in healthy people of the same age.

A deposit of beta-amyloid peptide (Aβ) stands out at the extracellular level. Aβ formations are also known as senile beta-amyloid plaques or simply amyloid plaques. However, at the intracellular level, an accumulation of hyperphosphorylated tau protein occurs; the latter is usually organized into clusters, which experts refer to as neurofibrillary tangles of hyperphosphorylated tau protein. It should be immediately noted that most likely the neurofibrillary bands of hyperphosphorylated tau protein are secondary to beta-amyloid plaques, that is, they result from the previous formation of the latter.

Aβ is a 36-43 amino acid peptide that is part of a larger protein known as amyloid precursor protein (APP).

APP is a trans membrane protein produced by neurons in the brain, the exact function of which is not yet known.

Beta-amyloid peptide originates from the initial proteolytic cleavage of APP by β-secretase and γ-secretase enzymes.

It then undergoes a process of enzymatic digestion under normal conditions, which causes its complete breakdown.

In patients with Alzheimer's disease, however, something different happens: partly for reasons that are not yet clear and partly for genetic reasons, the proteolytic cleavage process of APP occurs defectively and is interrupted during the formation of the beta-amyloid peptide; this interruption results in the accumulation of the Aβ peptide. Initially, there is an accumulation of soluble aggregates of beta-amyloid, while at the next stage, it produces large insoluble fragments, which subsequently precipitate, forming so-called "amyloid plaques."

There are several types of Aβ peptides: the best known and most common are Ap40 and Ap42.

Laboratory studies on brain slices have shown that amyloid plaques are neurotoxic; in particular, they damage synapses and cause the death of brain neurons. In addition, other studies have shown that they exhibit selective neurotoxicity to the hippocampus and entorhinal cortex; this evidence is particularly interesting given that the hippocampus and entorhinal cortex are regions of the brain most prone to atrophy in Alzheimer's patients.

Tau is an intracellular protein abundant in neurons and the central nervous system and plays an important role in stabilizing microtubules in the axons of nerve cells (particularly neurons).

In patients with Alzheimer's disease, abnormal deposition of hyperphosphorylated tau protein in the cell body of neurons is evident; in particular, tau pairs wrap around each other to form the aforementioned neurofibrillary bands.

Insoluble and abnormal accumulations of hyperphosphorylated tau in the cytoplasm displace intracellular organelles and change the distance between the microtubules with which they associate.

These changes in cellular microarchitecture lead to a change in axonal transport of substances that feed the axon terminal and the dendrites that generally keep the neuron alive. Genetic studies in Alzheimer's patients have shown that there are no mutations in the abnormal tau protein gene, leading experts to conclude that neurofibrillary tangles are independent of genetic factors.

Biochemistry

Beta-Amyloid plaques, specifically Aβ40 and Aβ42, cause the death of neurons, in fact related studies have shown that their aggregation has significant neurotoxic effects, specifically:

It blocks ion channels;

- Modifies calcium ion homeostasis;
- It increases oxidative stress at the mitochondrial level;
- It reduces energy metabolism;
- It affects glucose regulation.

The ultimate consequence of all these effects is a degeneration in the health of the neuron ending in its death.

In addition to the degeneration of neurons such Aβ plaques trigger the formation of neurofibrillary tangles, in fact, beta-amyloid deposits form soluble aggregates; then they give rise to insoluble clusters, which after their disintegration become true plaques characteristic of Alzheimer's disease.

Researchers have found that the massive formation of insoluble beta-amyloid plaques leads to the activation of certain protein kinases; upon activation, these protein kinases are responsible for hyper-phosphorylation of the microtubule-related tau protein. This process destabilizes the structure of tau protein and promotes its association with homologous protein until the formation of neurofibrillary bundles characteristic of Alzheimer's disease.

The accumulation of neurofibrillary tangles of tau protein impairs communication between neurons and affects axonal transport; in fact, the consequence of these effects is the death of the neurons themselves.

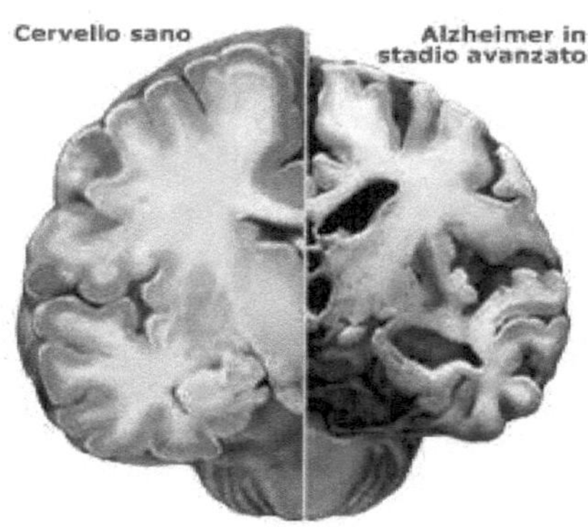

1.3 The various stages of Alzheimer's disease: symptoms and complications

First, it should be specified that there is the so-called 5-A disease, which correspond to the 5 cognitive disabilities common to all types of dementia: amnesia, aphasia, apraxia, agnosia, and anomia.

- Amnesia is memory loss and is often most evident when people with Alzheimer's disease begin to have difficulty with short-term memory, which eventually turns into long-term memory loss. As memory loss progresses, communication difficulties arise.
- Aphasia refers to communication disorders. The individual has difficulty understanding what is being said and difficulty expressing thoughts in words; he or she cannot find the right words or say them correctly.

- Apraxia is a loss of voluntary motor skills, so you lose the ability to perform daily tasks such as washing, dressing, walking and eating.
- Agnosia is the loss of the ability to recognize objects, faces, sounds, or places. The patient not only loses the ability to name an object, but also the ability to describe what it is for.
- Anomia is a situation in which the connection between neurons in the brain is weakened and it is difficult for the patient to find the right word. A person knows what object he needs and what he does, but he cannot find the right word.

Alzheimer's disease is a condition characterized by the gradual death of neurons in the brain; this phenomenon causes various stages to subsist and the symptoms consisting of neurological manifestations to gradually and inevitably worsen over time; therefore, the disease can be divided into four stages:

FIRST STAGE, lasting 1-3 years, characterized by symptoms and signs that are not always easy to recognize, often underestimated or misinterpreted as the cause of "passing years" such as stress, nervous exhaustion or too much work.
These are the following complications:
- difficulty in finding the right word to name objects or express concepts;
- difficulty remembering the date, time, meeting place and phone numbers;
- Changes in character and mood.

SECOND STAGE i.e., clear and obvious symptoms of the disease. Often this evidence appears due to the development of a "borderline" or already moderate cognitive state. This stage, also called moderate dementia, can last from 3 to 6 years and is characterized by the following symptoms and signs:

- difficulty in performing complex tasks, critical ability and abstract thinking apparently impaired, social difficulties;
- Temporal and often spatial disorientation;
- Difficulty remembering people's names;
- apraxia for complex direct movements.

THIRD STAGE lasting 2-3 years, characterized by progressive loss of functional ability in simple activities of daily living related to the following symptoms:

- Difficulty in recognizing relatives, friends, familiar objects;
- Loss of speech to the utterance of simple syllables or muteness;
- Frantic activity and/or constant vocalization;
- Progressive difficulty in walking with high risk of falls;
- Inability to leave the house, even if present;
- Urinary and fecal incontinence;
Reckless and/or strange behavior;
- Loss of functional autonomy in the simple activities of life

FOURTH STAGE or severe dementia lasting 1-2 years in which the person lives a vegetative life and is completely dependent on others. In particular we report:

- Complete inability to communicate even nonverbally;

- constraint to wheelchair use or full hospitalization with all the possible complications of immobilization syndrome (ulcers, infectious diseases...);

- total inability to eat and probable dysphagia with nasogastric gavage (NGS) or PEG. Apparently, malnutrition is the norm and the risk of dehydration is very high.

The onset of the disease takes an average of 10 to 12 years, although the variation can range from 2 to 20 years. However, there are cases in which the development is more rapid (death within 3 to 5 years of disease onset).

1.4 Patient risk factors

Some research has shown that important factors increase the likelihood of developing Alzheimer's disease. The most important of these risk conditions are:

- Age: Approximately one in twenty people with Alzheimer's disease will develop the disease above the age of 65. Recent data seem to suggest that age-related problems such as atherosclerosis may be important risk factors.

- Gender: Some studies show that the number of women with this disease has always been high compared with the number of men. However, this information may be misleading because women live longer on average than men.

- Genetic factors: On average, half of the children of a sick parent will inherit the disease, with onset at a relatively young age: usually between 35 and 60. A link between chromosome 21 and Alzheimer's disease has been discovered; since Down syndrome is caused by an abnormality on this chromosome, such individuals are more likely to become ill if they reach middle age, even if the full symptoms of the disease do not appear.

- Head trauma: there is good reason to believe that a person who has received a violent blow to the head may be at risk of getting Alzheimer's disease. The risk is higher if at the time of the blow the person is over fifty years old, has a specific gene (apoE4), and lost consciousness immediately after the blow.

2. MANAGEMENT OF THE ALZHEIMER'S PATIENT: A DROP OF MEMORY AS SOCIAL INTEGRATION

2.1 Non-pharmacological and psychosocial therapies

In addition to pharmacological treatments, drug-free treatment is widely used and effective. Indeed, they help patients maintain their cognitive abilities for as long as possible, promoting independence in daily activities, mental and physical well-being and social relationships. They also improve the control of psychological and behavioral symptoms such as restlessness, aggression and depression with positive effects on the patient's quality of life and the peace of mind of caregivers.

With the help of nonmedical care, it is possible:

- strengthen and improve cognitive and functional abilities, preserving those who are still ill or slowing their loss;

- Management of mental disorders and behavioral symptoms;

- Promotes disability compensation strategies;

- Promotes the maintenance of patients' functional autonomy including measures concerning their living environment;

- Promotes its social relations;

- Improves the quality of life for patients and their families

There are various types of interventions. The following are just a few of them.

- Cognitive interventions that aim at the cognitive well-being of the patient and are divided into 3 types:

- Cognitive training: the purpose is to strengthen certain cognitive functions such as memory, attention and language, which are impaired by the disease. .

- Cognitive rehabilitation: the goal is to strengthen the cognitive skills and processes needed to perform daily tasks important to a person, thereby reducing the disability of the disease and protecting the function, efficiency, and independence of sufferers.

- Cognitive stimulation: the goal is to improve a person's overall cognitive and social functioning and to engage in enjoyable and meaningful activities, often in a group setting.

- Reminiscence therapy

This activity aims to refresh patients' autobiographical memory and preserve vivid memories of life experiences that may be obscured by cognitive decline. It can be done individually or in groups and uses visual and auditory stimuli such as photos, music, videos and objects to help people recall past events and feelings.

- Pet therapy procedures

Pet therapy procedures also aim to improve the well-being, mental and physical health and quality of life of patients in cooperation with specially trained pets. In general, this intervention can benefit the elderly as it stimulates movement and has a positive effect on mood.

- Doll Therapy

Doll therapy is designed to alleviate behavioral symptoms in people with Alzheimer's disease, especially the severe forms. It is based on the treatment of a doll, which must have certain characteristics and be given to the patient in precise ways to remind him or her deeply of the instinctive relationship between mother and child. The positive effects of doll therapy include reduction of aggression and anxiety and better control of disorders such as wandering.

- The Snoezelen Approach

Originating in the Netherlands in the 1970s, the Snoezelen approach aims to promote human well-being through guided multisensory stimulation in a specific environment: the "Snoezelen Room." It was originally developed for people with severe intellectual disabilities, but over time it has also proven effective in the treatment of diseases such as Alzheimer's disease and dementia. It is therefore, through this space, that the approach to the person becomes an entirely nonmedical treatment. In people with Alzheimer's disease and dementia, it is used as a therapeutic intervention to encourage stimulation of the five senses through visual, tactile, sound, taste and smell effects; it requires no special cognitive skills, only the use of sensory and motor skills.

The Snoezelen Room can help foster relationships, encourage participation or relaxation, and prevent or reduce behavioral problems in Alzheimer's disease such as restlessness, depression, and aggression. Based on studies, this approach also appears to have the ability to improve the mood of dementia patients and help them interact more easily with their caregivers and their environment.

- Motor rehabilitation

Alzheimer's disease is a neurodegenerative disease that primarily causes cognitive impairment, but can also have motor effects. This results in difficulties with posture, problems with walking and balance, and difficulties with fine hand movements, such as those requiring precision and hand-eye coordination, such as tying shoes. It is therefore helpful to provide a motor rehabilitation program appropriate to the patient's needs and the severity of the condition. In the early stage, physiotherapeutic intervention should aim to slow the progression of Alzheimer's disease and prevent the negative physical development of the disease through a general fitness program. Regular physical activity is beneficial in improving cardiovascular health in patients with dementia, which is less correlated with brain degeneration.

In advanced stages, the goal of motor stimulation should be to help the patient maintain motor skills to the best of his or her ability.

- Speech therapy rehabilitation

Alzheimer's disease and dementia often require speech therapy to treat speech and swallowing disorders. Problems in the area of communication-language strongly affect the patient's quality of life and can contribute to social isolation and loss of self-esteem. These include difficulties related to oral and written expression and speech articulation, such as aphasia, dysarthria and dysphonia as well as sensory disorders such as hearing loss, hearing loss, especially quiet or distant sounds or words.

In people with neurodegenerative diseases, these difficulties are often accompanied by dysphagia, a swallowing disorder that, if left untreated, can lead to serious health risks, especially malnutrition. Therefore, it is important to provide speech rehabilitation therapy with interventions aimed at preventing and treating these problems.

2.2 Drug treatment

Many therapeutic strategies have been viewed for several decades; however, there is still no curative treatment for this disease, and the priority remains prevention. In any case, drugs used in therapy can relieve symptoms or otherwise prolong the timing of the first and second stages of Alzheimer's disease.

There are four molecules currently approved and available in Italy for the treatment of Alzheimer's disease: donepezil, rivastigmine, galantamine, and memantine, in order of approval. The first three are approved for mild and moderate forms, memantine for moderate and severe forms. Since 2002 (approval of memantine), no new drugs have been clinically reviewed or approved for treatment of the disease.

The availability of molecules, although they share a common mechanism of action, allows better tailoring of therapy with different pharmacological, pharmacokinetic, pharmacometabolic profiles and dosage forms, as with many other drug classes. The GP, as with other treatments, may be more familiar with one of these. The main side effects associated with excessive cholinergic activation are similar for the three drugs.

Memantine, approved for the treatment of moderate to severe forms of Alzheimer's disease, is a noncompetitive NMDA (N-methyl-D-aspartate) glutamate receptor antagonist. The drug is believed to limit excessive basal glutamatergic activity, which promotes neurodegeneration and makes transmission less efficient.

Memantine has long been used in Europe as an anti-aging brain drug, after which it was registered for the treatment of Alzheimer's disease after an ad hoc clinical trial. A molecule with different class and mechanism of action, it is useful because it offers an alternative for patients who do not respond to acetylcholinesterase inhibitors.

Some patients also have the option of combining an acetylcholinesterase inhibitor with memantine therapy.

Various authors have tested and proposed a link between the two drugs, although no consensus has been reached on their efficacy. It should be remembered that two different acetylcholinesterase inhibitors cannot be combined because of the sum of side effects.

Another advantage of the different drugs is that they have a different side effect profile than acetylcholinesterase inhibitors.

But what do you get out of the available medications? Drugs can keep symptoms under control for a while, after which progression continues. We are not far from ideal, but this is an effect also recognized in international guidelines. The physician, together with the nurse, should know the limitations of current treatment methods and, after starting it, explain them to the patient and family members. It is also worth clarifying that not all patients have an efficient response to drug treatment.

All other medications taken by the patient should also be considered, especially those used to treat behavioral disorders (anxiety, depression, psychotic disorders, delusions). It should be emphasized immediately that medication should generally be avoided for behavioral control and that nonpharmacological forms of intervention should be preferred whenever possible. If a decision is made to use medication, its actual need should be carefully monitored, starting with the smallest doses and carefully monitoring the occurrence of possible side effects. Finally, all other drugs used for very common diseases related to aging should be considered. General considerations here relate to the criteria for suitability of prescription for elderly patients, as well as to the maintenance of the sedative effect at anticholinergic load and possible interactions of various drugs provided.

2.3 Nursing care for patients with dementia

The goal of nursing care for patients with Alzheimer's disease is to maintain good functioning and independence for as long as possible. Helping the individual through physical safety, anxiety reduction, independence in daily self-care activities, improved communication, adequate intimacy, proper nutrition, and caregiver education are important.

In the early stage of the disease, a person can maintain reasonable autonomy, such that he or she does not need constant help; however, as the disease progresses,

receives more help from formal caregivers, e.g., health workers and informal caregivers, e.g., relatives It is recommended that a quiet environment without excessive noise for the patient should always be ensured; the daily routine should be regular and communication should be through small and simple dialogues.

The patient should be encouraged to always be active both mentally and physically: in fact, regular physical activity and socialization have been shown to reduce and slow the progression of the disease. In particular, exercise improves the sleep-wake rhythm, which AD tends to balance.

As the disease progresses, simple daily activities become difficult and often impossible; therefore, they must be organized in such a way that the patient is able to perform them. Loss of independence and the ability to stop doing things that were previously possible can make a person anxious or agitated, especially during times of awareness, lucidity, and cognitive decline. In these cases, it is advisable to approach the person calmly and patiently and look for an activity that can distract and calm him or her.

It is not uncommon for a patient to scream, cry or become verbally and physically aggressive. In this regard, training for health care professionals is essential: family members must actually be able to recognize these behaviors and be able to decipher them.

Nurses and all other health care workers play a vital role; in fact, they not only have to support the patient, but they also carry a considerable emotional burden. It is difficult to cope with the fact that one of their loved ones has a diagnosis of Alzheimer's, as it is a progressive and degenerative disease with no cure, family members watch the patient's progressive deterioration without being able to do anything. They often misinterpret some of the patient's behaviors or attitudes and become unable to help.

In Italy, there are associations of family members and professionals, such as the Italian Alzheimer's Association and Alzheimer's Association Italy, that provide support and assistance to both patients and their families.

2.4 The importance of the caregiver in the emotional management of the patient

The patient's family members, who first feel the early signs of the disease and experience the first discomforts related to it, play a key role in raising awareness of the disease and

often do not know what to do. Therefore, institutions must provide the right psychological and medical support.

Pathological forms that cause a progressive deterioration of personality abilities and independence, such as dementia, lead to a radical change in living conditions, both on a practical-behavioral and emotional level.Thus, Alzheimer's disease is a disease that affects not just one person, but the whole family. In most cases, it is the family that takes care of the home care of the sick person.

Family members face many changes. On the one hand, there are organizational changes in terms of time spent monitoring, managing, and reconciling other work responsibilities; on the other hand, the management of social relations outside the family changes. The environment, understood in its broader human and relational context, must also be adapted to the patient in such a way that he or she can maintain residual functional capacities for as long as possible and limit the aggravation of behavioral disorders.

Moreover, in the context of this encounter, psychological factors come into play for the family member, who has to deal with the suffering and anxiety caused by the feeling of loss and helplessness, and with the difficulty of understanding what is happening to the person who, until recently, represented the emotional and relational "pillar" of the family itself.

Over time, awareness of the reality of the disease grows. The family rationally understands that there is no miracle drug. What does exist, however, is a disease that, in addition to pain and confusion, can cause severe anxiety related to the "need" to be constantly busy. The need to be constantly alert and active underlies the need not to think too much about the situation one is experiencing. Coping with a patient's difficulties every day can be very painful. To avoid such suffering and to protect the patient from failure, the family member often tends to constantly protect the patient and be very empathetic.

It happens very often that the feeling of anger is replaced by another painful experience: guilt. There are many reasons that can make a family member feel guilty: loss of patience, shame about the patient's condition and behavior, recollection of some conflict situation with him, a desire for everything to end.

Family members' awareness of this feeling, which is common to all people with Alzheimer's disease, is important because it can help them recognize and accept their limitations in living with the disease.

As the disease progresses over time, the family realizes that the constant investment of energy to bring the patient back to a "normal" state will not succeed. This then leads to intense frustration, which often turns to anger. The sick person's behavior is actually not intentional, but is a manifestation of the symptoms of the disease.

If one encounters a moment of anger or difficulty in general, it is advisable to seek help, turn to experts, and share one's experiences and doubts with others who have gone through or are going through similar experiences. However, the process of accepting the illness consists of the difficulties that the patient faces and the changes that these critical issues inevitably bring about, both on a family and personal level. The result of this process is the restructuring of family dynamics and organizational and communication arrangements that must become functional in the patient's home care. Indeed, the task of helping is a very demanding one and requires constant acceptance of the patient's feelings. Therefore, the family member must prevent the illness from becoming the center of his or her life.

3. ARTIFICIAL INTELLIGENCE AS A NEW METHOD OF DIAGNOSIS

3.1 Current research and prevention studies in dementia

The concept of dementia prevention is of relatively recent origin and stands in stark contrast to the pessimistic view traditionally associated with age-related diseases in both the general population and a significant proportion of health care professionals. This still prevalent negative attitude may be based on the classic biological concept of "neuronal loss," which occurs in normal aging and in an accelerated and accentuated form in age-related degenerative diseases. Apparent interindividual differences in cognitive function in old age, according to this strictly deterministic view, depend only and primarily, on nonvariable factors, such as genetic inheritance.

The possibility of prevention is closely linked to the development of the concept of 'brain plasticity' that is, the structural and functional variability of the brain based on environmental factors and experiences.

In the case of Alzheimer's disease, the share of potentially modifiable factors in the development of dementia is estimated to be 35 percent. There are nine main factors: low educational level, high blood pressure and obesity at intermediate stages, deafness, depression in the elderly, diabetes, sedentary lifestyle, smoking and social isolation. Of course, the items that make up the list are not a surprise to the physician, but perhaps surprising is the magnitude of their contribution. In the case of a disease with such a large epidemiologic impact, there is an opportunity to reduce or, in any case, delay the onset of clinical symptoms at the level of primary or secondary prevention. A key concept is cognitive reserve. The onset of the clinical syndrome of dementia is only one manifestation of the process of organ failure that develops in the brain; in fact, in Alzheimer's disease, the progressive deterioration of synaptic function and death of neurons is due to a complex sequence of pathogenic events. This process begins several years before the onset of clinical symptoms, the appearance of which indicates that a critical threshold of damage to organ function has been exceeded.

It is crucial to make a difference between brain resistance and resilience. The concept of cognitive reserve is formed in the mechanisms of "resilience," that is, the ability to adapt to the onset and progression of neuropathology. These include: brain reserve, i.e., individual differences in brain structure, which may contribute to a better ability to "absorb" the burden of pathology; cognitive reserve or ability to compensate for the impact of pathology through functional reorganization of the brain; and "brain maintenance," which refers to changes in both structural and functional parameters of the brain over time. Along with these compensatory mechanisms, possible individual differences in resistance to pathology should be considered, resulting in their absence or reduced expression. From a practical point of view, there is a fundamental difference between the incremental factors of resistance and resilience that are modifiable and those that are not. At this stage, the theoretical concepts developed so far are combined with epidemiology, which has revealed risk factors and protective factors for Alzheimer's disease. This information forms the basis for preventive research, which must answer the fundamental question of clinical practice, namely, whether intervention in risk groups can be effective, if possible. For example, physical activity could reduce the risk of cognitive decline in old age, and this comes from studies in which subjects provided information about their "lifestyles," that is, choices and behaviors that may be characteristic of people associated then with other elements of a "healthy lifestyle" and often with ethnic and cultural factors (a typical example is the Mediterranean diet). A clinically important question is whether implementing a change, usually later in life, can lead to a reduction in risk in individuals who previously followed a different, less "protective" lifestyle. The evidence from various studies and research has become largely true, and the results are encouraging.

3.2 How to diagnose Alzheimer's disease

The diagnosis of Alzheimer's disease is based on several studies, since there is still no specific test to detect the disease, it is essential to get help from several specialists, including psychiatrists, neurologists, and geriatricians; in addition, statements from the patient's relatives are important, compensating for the patient's own difficulties in explaining the symptoms and disorders that affect him or her.

The diagnosis of Alzheimer's disease also involves an exclusion approach: this is the so-called 'differential diagnosis,' which includes tests and examinations aimed at ruling out the possibility that current symptoms are caused by other diseases.

In general, the diagnosis of Alzheimer's disease is based on the following data:

- Medical history;
- Physical examination;
- Neurological examination;
- Cognitive and neuropsychological testing;
- Laboratory tests;
- Diagnostic imaging studies involving the brain.

A medical history, also called a medical history, is the collection of any information from the direct voice of the patient and/or family that is useful in explaining a particular symptom. It usually includes questions about the patient's general health status, habits, lifestyle, treatment modalities followed, any previous illnesses, and family medical history. When diagnosing Alzheimer's disease, the medical history is important because it provides insight into whether current symptoms are actually caused by the dementia in question.

Objective examination or physical examination consists of a medical assessment of the patient's general health status. It provides diagnostic procedures used by a physician to confirm the presence or absence of signs of a specific disease condition. Objective examination is a mandatory step in the diagnosis of any disease, including Alzheimer's disease, although it alone is not sufficient for definitive conclusions.

The neurological examination assesses tendon reflexes, motor skills (e.g., balance, coordination...) and sensory function. In the diagnosis of Alzheimer's disease, a neurological examination can be considered a more thorough objective examination that deepens the knowledge of the patient's health status.

Cognitive and neuropsychological testing tests the patient on various fronts and abilities such as memory, problem-solving ability, language and communication skills, reasoning and calculation skills, and finally behavioral and psychiatric functioning.

Cognitive and neuropsychological examination can provide very useful diagnostic information, sometimes decisive in confirming the pathology; However, it is good to specify the importance of its application, because always take into account certain aspects of the patient, such as the patient's level of education and general physical health (level of hearing, vision, etc.) as they may distort the patient's result.

Cognitive tests are used not only for diagnostic purposes but also to assess the progression and severity of Alzheimer's disease. One cognitive test particularly suitable for diagnosing Alzheimer's disease is the Mini-Mental Test, also known as the Mini-Mental State Examination or Folstein test. The Mini-Mental Test is a 30-question questionnaire that allows one to analyze one's calculations, memory, reasoning, language and attention on a person.

The Mini-Mental Status Examination is useful for diagnosing all dementias, not just Alzheimer's disease.

In addition, the diagnosing physician wants to use special laboratory tests to analyze various parameters, of the blood (but not only) whose alterations are usually accompanied by symptoms that may resemble those of Alzheimer's disease. Thus, laboratory tests are used from the point of view of differential diagnosis: they help to exclude diseases and conditions characterized by symptomatology overlapping with Alzheimer's disease, which can be confused with the latter.

Useful laboratory tests to diagnose Alzheimer's disease include those of blood glucose, measurement of vitamin B12 in the blood, urinalysis, toxicology test (indicates whether or not symptoms are due to consumption of a drug or other toxic substance), and blood test for thyroid hormones.

Brain CT and MRI brain scans provide detailed three-dimensional images.

Similar to laboratory tests, CT and MRI are used in differential diagnosis-they are not really specific tests for Alzheimer's disease, but they can detect brain diseases such as strokes, tumors, and vascular disorders that cause symptoms similar to the aforementioned dementia.

Some variants of PET (positron emission tomography) can identify amyloid plaques, neurofibrillary tangles of tau protein, and other signs of brain degeneration characteristic of Alzheimer's disease, however, it is important to note that these methods are used in disease research and clinical trials, not in routine diagnosis.

In addition, when Alzheimer's disease is diagnosed through differential diagnosis, other conditions such as Parkinson's disease, sleep disorders, side effects of drugs or toxic substances, and aging-related cognitive decline are ruled out regardless.

Therefore, the so-called early diagnosis of Alzheimer's disease (AD) using biomarkers is also useful, which can help implement and monitor early therapeutic interventions and can significantly change the course of the disease.

Classic cerebrospinal fluid and approved structural and functional neuroimaging biomarkers have limited clinical use because of their invasive nature and/or high cost. Identifying biomarkers that are easier to use and cheaper are blood biomarkers would increase their use in clinical practice. Blood biomarkers are more cost and time efficient than cerebrospinal fluid biomarkers. However, immediate use in clinical practice is relatively unlikely. The main limitations stem from difficulties in measuring and standardizing threshold values among different laboratories and the inability to reproduce results. Of all the molecules studied, biomarkers of apoptosis and neurodegeneration obtained by "omics" approaches such as isolated or combined metabolomics provide the most promising results.

3.3 Artificial intelligence for health.

Artificial intelligence (AI) is a modern computer science-based approach that develops programs and algorithms that make devices intelligent and efficient in performing tasks that normally require skilled human intelligence. AI includes several subsets such as machine learning (ML), deep learning (DL), conventional neural networks, fuzzy logic, and speech recognition, which have unique features and functions that can improve the efficiency of modern medicine. Such intelligent systems facilitate human intervention in clinical diagnosis, medical imaging and decision making. Meanwhile, the Internet of Medical Things (IoMT) is emerging as a next-generation bioanalytic tool that connects online biomedical devices with software to improve human health. As with all technological innovations, it is important to make safety and risk management considerations.

Therefore, recognizing the great potential of artificial intelligence to accelerate the digital transformation of health care, the World Health Organization (WHO) lists the most important regulations in a new publication, 'Regulatory considerations on Artificial Intelligence for health,' which aims to promote its safe, effective and responsible use in the health sector.

The document, which provides guidance to authorities on artificial intelligence in health, is part of WHO's Global Strategy for Digital Health 2020-2025, which aims to improve human health at any age by developing and implementing appropriate, accessible, affordable, scalable, sustainable, and human-centered digital technologies for disease prevention, detection, and response.

WHO points out that artificial intelligence in healthcare offers many opportunities by preventing disease; diagnosing, treating and monitoring the delivery of health services to disadvantaged populations; improving public health surveillance; promoting health research and drug development; supporting the management of health systems under pressure; and enabling professionals to make complex medical diagnoses to improve care and treatment options.

However, existing and emerging artificial intelligence technologies, including large language models, are often used without a full understanding of how such systems work and the potential benefits or harms to end users, including health care providers and patients.

Therefore, the WHO, together with the International Telecommunication Union (ITU), created the FG-AI4H to facilitate the safe and appropriate use of artificial intelligence and to ensure the protection of sensitive data and the security of all healthcare stakeholders.

WHO has identified six key areas to define AI health regulation:

- Documentation and transparency: to promote trust, WHO stresses the importance of transparency and documentation, such as documenting the entire product life cycle and monitoring development processes;
- Life cycle risk management and artificial intelligence system development: from a risk management perspective, issues such as use continuous learning, human intervention, training models, and cybersecurity threats need to be comprehensive and dealt with using simpler models;
- Intended use and analytical and clinical validation: external data validation and clarity of the intended use of AI help ensure safety and facilitate regulation;
- Data quality: ensuring data quality, such as through rigorous evaluation of systems before publication, is important to ensure that systems do not introduce bias or errors;
- Privacy and data protection: challenges arising from important and complex regulations such as GDPR in Europe and HIPAA (Health Insurance Portability and Accountability Act) in America need to be addressed, paying particular attention to the fact that the scope of jurisdiction and consent requirements for privacy and data protection;
- Involvement and collaboration: fostering collaboration among regulators, patients, health care providers, industry and government

partners can help ensure compliance of products and services throughout their lifecycle.

3.4 AI as a possible weapon for prevention and diagnostics.

Artificial intelligence (AI) in medical laboratories may be the right support in preventing Alzheimer's disease, the most common form of dementia. A recent study published in the Journal of Alzheimer's Disease explains how new analytical methods related to neurodegenerative diseases such as Alzheimer's disease can help detect its occurrence through the power of artificial intelligence.

The study, conducted by researchers from the University of Chieti-Pescara, the University of Irvine and the University of California, San Francisco, used a huge international database that collects information on thousands of patients with neurodegenerative diseases and combined it with machine learning, a model developed by biotechnology experts. Professor Stefano Sensi, director of the Dnisci Department of Neuroscience, Imaging Sciences and Clinical Sciences at Chieti University, and Professor Stefano Sensi, director of the Cast Advanced Research and Technology Center, coordinated the mechanisms involved in the research. On the development of Alzheimer's disease and the possibility of early diagnosis of the disease that indicates new hope for treatment. The study focused specifically on analyzing the value of extra- and intra-cerebral factors in creating the transition from an early and potentially treatable condition (mild cognitive impairment) to dementia. "The algorithm we developed analyzed hundreds of brain, neuropsychological, cerebrospinal fluid and blood data collected from patients in the international database Adni (Alzheimer's Disease Neuroimaging Initiative)," Sensi explained. In particular, experts were surprised that artificial intelligence could highlight the possibility of non-brain factors, including, for example, changes in the concentrations of certain bile acids and underlying neurodegenerative processes. A factor consistent with the process of the "gut-brain connection," that is, the correlation between the nervous system and the gastrointestinal tract. As Davide Nardini and Giorgio Maria Mandolini, the experts who developed the algorithm, point out, "Thanks to the use of new variables identified by artificial intelligence, the model achieved 98 percent accuracy in some cases." According to the researchers, among other things, "the fields of medicine and bioinformatics have many imaginable applications and will become very common in the coming years-a good reason to invest capital and knowledge in this field," they say.

The latest developments in artificial intelligence in relation to language and particularly in speech recognition (Speech Recognition), natural language processing (NAT), and speech synthesis (TTS) have paved the way for new possibilities in health and prevention of various diseases and/or illnesses.

Already in 2018, voice recordings of healthy people and people with dementia were analyzed in several studies. The AI algorithm was able to accurately identify the presence of dementia in 89% of cases. Another 2019 study used a speech recognition system to examine voice characteristics such as speed and pitch and predict the likelihood of developing dementia.

Using speech as a biomarker could provide a rapid, inexpensive, accurate and noninvasive diagnosis of Alzheimer's disease and other forms of dementia.

In addition, voice assistants have been widely used during pandemics, such as in France, where the technology supported patients with COVID-19. Since then, several healthcare features have been added to Amazon's Alexa, Apple's Siri and Google's Home Assistant to provide assistance to patients remotely.

Advances in speech technology, audio signal analysis, and natural language processing and understanding methods have thus paved the way for many potential audio applications, such as detection of auditory biomarkers for diagnosis, remote monitoring of patients, and improvement of clinical practice.

In the context of voice, a voice biomarker, like a signature, is a combination of features associated with a clinical outcome that can be used to monitor patients, diagnose a condition or classify the severity or stages of a disease or manage it.

Subtle changes in voice and speech can often be detected years before Alzheimer's symptoms appear and can be detected in the early stages of cognitive decline.

In general, cognitive impairment affects verbal fluency, which is manifested by the patient's hesitation to speak and slowing of speech speed. Other indicators include word-finding difficulties leading to repeated use of filler vowels, semantic errors, undefined terms, versions, repetitions, neologisms, lexical and grammatical simplifications, and a general loss of semantic skills.

Changes are also observed in prosody--variation and modulation of tone, rhythm of speech--and may affect the patient's emotional reactivity.

Linguistic modeling (LM) is the use of various statistical techniques to determine the probability that a given set of words will occur to decide. Language models are used in various applications that typically produce text such as machine translation, question answering, and summarizing.

Among the many language models that have appeared for their high efficiency are the American OpenAI GPT models of the Microsoft Group. GPT stands for generative pre-training because this family of models is trained in two separate steps, the first (pre-training) simply consists of "predicting the next word" on a huge set of documents; the second step is the guided fine-tuning of certain tasks, such as answering questions or classifying text. This type of training provides a very versatile model, while, because of the huge amount of data it uses, it can produce text that is almost indistinguishable from text written by humans.

A study by Agbavori and Liang in 2022 used recordings from the ADReSSo (Alzheimer's Dementia Detection through Spontaneous Speech Only) challenge, converted them to text using speech synthesis techniques, applied GPT 2 and GPT-3 language models, and succeeded in obtaining an important result. These language models seem to be even better in predicting dementia than voice analysis and voice biomarkers.

The research is just beginning, and the field is clearly new and thus requires all attention, diligence and especially care. However, these are interesting results that offer hope for improving the prevention

of neurodegenerative diseases such as Alzheimer's and other forms
of dementia.

4. TECHNOLOGICAL INNOVATIONS FOR THE FUTURE OF THE HEALTH CARE SYSTEM

4.1 The evolution of AI: the use of new artificial neural networks

The term "artificial neural network" or in English " artificial neural network" refers to a mathematical model in the field of machine learning that aims to resemble the biological neural networks that exist in humans or animals and that consists of artificial neurons constructed virtually or sometimes physically. The purpose of this technology is to help solve computer problems and especially those related to the field of artificial intelligence in the field of medicine. In order to find increasingly precise solutions, neural networks are trained with different types of machine learning, which vary depending on the purpose for which they are produced.

First of all, it is essential to analyze a neuron in its totality. A neuron present in our brain is composed of the soma i.e., the cell body in which the nucleus is inserted from which the dendrites emerge, an axon (also connected to the cell body but thicker and more robust than the dendrites) and the axon endings. We have to imagine that in our brain there is a real network consisting of hundreds of millions of neurons made up of this same structure.

What happens for the biological neuron is that the moment an impulse arrives through the dendrites, the cell body is charged with electricity, it acts as a kind of capacitor and accumulates the electrical charges, but clearly, the soma has a limit of accumulation, and so once it reaches the maximum amount of electrical energy it can accumulate, the axon comes into play. The latter acts as an outflow channel; the cell body discharges the electrical energy into the axon. This, in turn, will transport that energy to the dendrites of another neuron. This dynamic of passing the electrical impulse from the axon to the dendrites is called a synapse.

In this way our brain is able to process enormous amounts of information: its peculiarity lies in the fact that the synapse is able to occur by activating numerous areas and does so simultaneously, such a mechanism is multiple and simultaneous.

Computers, on the other hand, work by processing data sequentially, performing one task at a time and then moving on to the next, and they do this in only one place at a time. It was for this very reason that those in the computer science field were interested in the opportunity to reproduce the biological system in an entirely artificial creation, so they tried to mimic the natural pattern of neurons, how a neural network works, and why this kind of technology was needed.

Considering the structure of a biological neural network, an attempt was made to reproduce in a simplified way a similar system that could work equally well in computing.

An artificial neural network consists of nodes or formal neurons, which are the basic computational units and which, when connected together, form a graph consisting of at least one input layer and one output layer. The purpose of this network is also to process data and information and it works on the input (which can be compared to the electrical impulse of a biological neuron) that arrives at the node of the input layer.

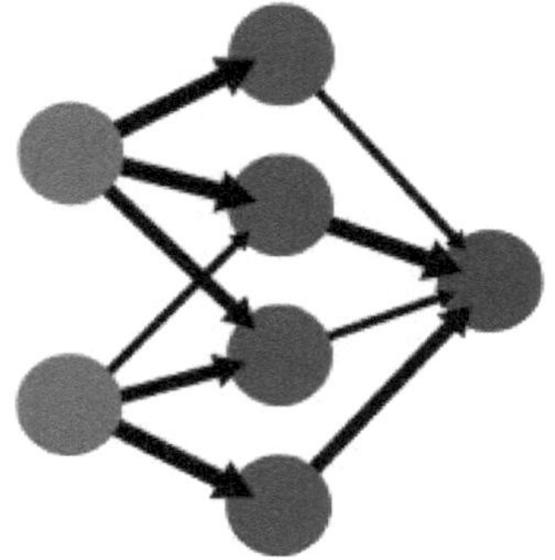

At this point, maintaining the basic operating principle, the artificial neuron is activated by this input and also receives the maximum "stimulus." Each node has a threshold value above which the received information is forwarded to the output layer. Somewhat like what happens between a cell body and an axon, when a certain amount of stored energy is exceeded, it is loaded into the axon and then onto another nearby neuron. The difference here is that the information is transmitted in the form of numbers, which are transmitted using mathematical functions.

At this stage, the data initially submitted are processed.

To ensure the effectiveness of this mechanism and thus the accurate processing of data, machine learning or, more precisely, deep learning methods are being studied, which train the neural network by making it perform better and better. The more you train a neural network, the better the algorithm will evolve to perform better.

From the 1950s to the present, different types of neural networks have been constructed; in fact, this topic has been studied for over 70 years!

Below we examine the different types of neural networks in use today:

- The first of all examples is the perceptron, a neural network created by psychologist Frank Rosenblatt in 1958, which basically consists of a single node receiving input and processing it through a function and then returning an output;

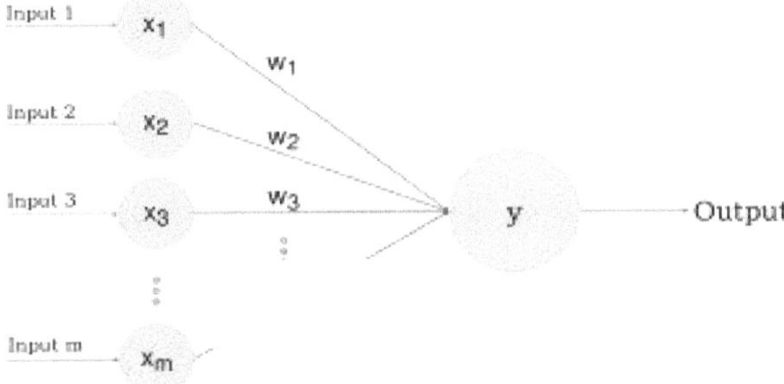

- Then there are feed forward networks, which are characterized by a unidirectional flow of information. They are divided into single-layer networks, when there is only one input layer and one output layer, and multilayer networks, when there are multiple intermediate layers of nodes that remain "hidden."

In the case of multilayer networks, because there are hidden layers, we are talking about deep neural networks trained with deep learning algorithms;

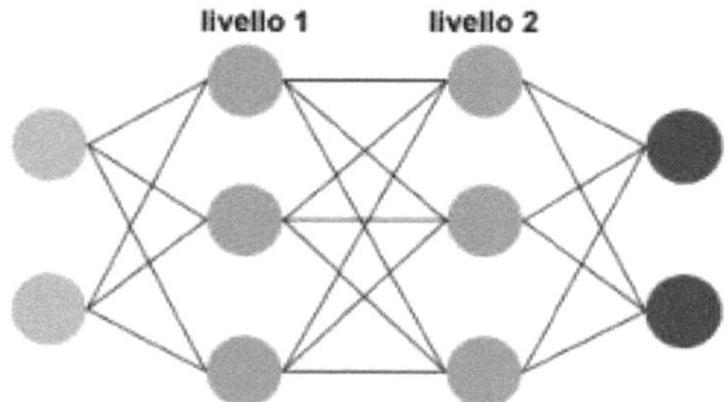

- The third type is Recurrent Neural Networks (RNNs), which are actually multilayer networks in which signals from the higher-level nodes, however, become inputs to the lower-level layers. In general, such a mechanism uses the output of one layer as the input of a lower layer to create a memory in the same network;

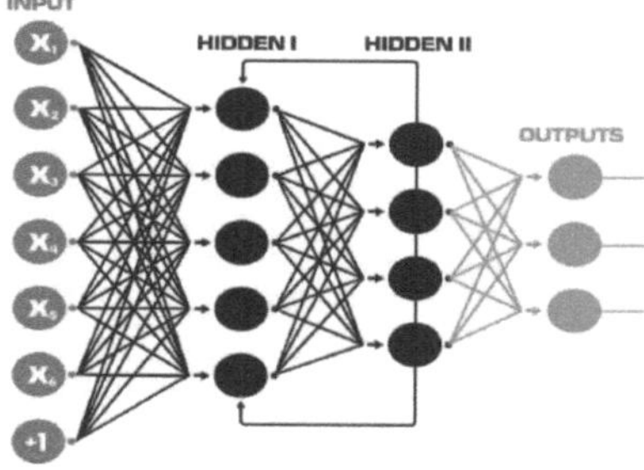

Image source: Geopop

- A final, even more complex type is Convolutional Neural Networks (CNN or ConvNet). They are actually a type of multilayer broadcast network consisting of at least five different layers (an input, a series of hidden layers, and an output).

44

Some of these hidden layers are called "convolutional layers," which perform a specific computer operation to build a true map of the input features obtained from the previous layer. This map is used as additional information to be added to the next layer for a very accurate and detailed printout. Being a very complex, multilayer neural network, it is trained with deep learning algorithms and used to process more complex data.

Neural network structures can be used very successfully in many fields, especially when large amounts of data are available for nodes to process as input. The best known use cases are image recognition (e.g., recognizing the face of the same person in several different images), as well as speech or text recognition.

Among the many areas of application for this technology are marketing, financial forecasting, food quality control, medical diagnostics, cybersecurity systems, license plates and banknotes, energy consumption forecasting, and more. Depending on the task at hand, each neural network is trained with a specific type of learning, ranging from as simple as machine learning to more sophisticated deep learning techniques.

It is certain that research on these aspects related to the world of artificial intelligence is still in its infancy, and often we do not even realize how many different aspects of daily life can bear fruit for the application of these new technologies.

4.2 First artificial neuron on microchip to fight Alzheimer's disease

As with coronary arteries, bypass will also come for synapses in the brain. In this case, however, it will help them replace functions lost due to brain cell death caused by neurodegenerative diseases such as Alzheimer's. We are talking about a hundred billion neurons, each of which is connected to ten thousand others: the brain's network of connections is in fact enormous, and unfortunately, as we get older, it can "tear apart" at some point, leading to more or less severe cognitive difficulties. Thanks to its plasticity, the brain compensates for the death of neurons for a long time, but when a certain threshold of damage is exceeded this is impossible and the symptoms of dementia appear. In the not too distant future, holes in the network of brain connections could be filled, or rather "bypassed" by synthetic neurons on chips: they already exist and have already been tested in vitro and on rats. These chips are analog, like the human body, receiving and transmitting electrical information like human neurons, but they cannot be controlled from the outside. They consume a billion times less energy than a normal microprocessor, so much so that they can use the microcurrents produced by biological neurons and do not require power. Today the chip is five millimeters square, but in the near future it may reach the diameter of a hair and can be implanted in damaged areas of the human brain and at least partially restore communication between cells and thus cognitive function. The results achieved and future prospects will be presented and discussed at an invitation-only conference organized by the Dementia Research Association Onlus at the 16th SIN-DEM (Autonomous Association Following SIN for Dementia) Congress.

"Neurons on chips are already a reality," explains professor and researcher in computer science and cybernetics Claude Kanah, "Today's microchips are small squares with an area of five millimeters square, and in the future they may be reduced to the diameter of a hair to be transplanted into the human brain. So far these artificial neurons have been tested in vitro on cultured neurons and, in vivo, in rats, where they were transplanted into critical areas such as the hippocampus, a region of the brain key to memory processes and less active in neurodegenerative diseases such as Alzheimer's. Experiments so far have shown that these silicon (i.e., artificial) neurons behave like biological ones: in other words, they respond to changes in electrical currents in the brain, and can transmit this information to other neurons in the form of electrical impulses."

The neurons in the chips could thus act as a "bridge" to repair a broken or damaged connection. Alain Nogaret of the University of Bath, Elisa Donati and Giacomo Indiveri of the University of Zurich and other researchers have so far conducted experiments in animals. Researchers from the Universities of Bristol and Auckland show that these solid-state neurons are able to behave like biological neurons and respond almost identically to many different stimuli. In addition, bionic neurons require very little power to operate, only 140 nanowatts, or about one billionth of the power required by a standard microprocessor.

"This means that they are simple and controllable systems because they can use the small currents generated continuously and physiologically by biological neurons for their operation: the goal is to make sure that the neurons on the chip receive their current at a low level. The power supply adapts to physiological feedbacks in real time and activates autonomously immediately after they are deployed, exploiting the electrical potential of existing neuronal networks," stresses Claudio Mariani, president of ARD Onlus and professor of neurology at the Sacco Hospital in Milan. "Moreover, these systems work with an analog and therefore continuous technology, not binary like the digital one: all biological systems are based on continuous processes, and choosing this strategy means being able to mimic even more closely the behavior of a biological neuron. Today we know that these neuromorphic processors can communicate with biological neurons because they "speak" the same language, which consists of electrical signals; the next step will be to test them, for example, in mice with genetically engineered Alzheimer's disease, to see if they can replace the functions of damaged neurons and how they can improve memory performance.

In fact, we can be very optimistic about the timing of human trials: when neuromorphic chips find a place in the human brain, they will interact with it and repair circuits damaged by neurodegenerative diseases. "The speed of progress in cybernetic sciences, which develops in the square of time" - concludes Leonardo Pantoni, vice president of ARD onlus, director and professor of the Department of Complex Neurology at Luigi Sacco Hospital in Milan. Neurology of the University of Milan - probably, in the next 5-10 years we will not only have a functional artificial neuron transplanted into the human brain, but also networks of artificial neurons that can be transplanted, for example, into areas affected by amyloid plaques in Alzheimer's disease or other degenerative diseases, working in parallel with other circuits and helping biological neurons to continue to perform their tasks.

4.3 Artificial intelligence in healthcare: more doctor-patient relationship and fewer errors in treatment

According to a study by GE Healthcare and MIT MIT-Technology Review Insights, the use of artificial intelligence enables healthcare workers to spend more time on human relationships, reduce medication errors and improve workflow.

The robust implementation of artificial intelligence in healthcare facilities brings numerous benefits. Seventy-eight percent of healthcare workers say the implementation of artificial intelligence solutions will improve their workflow, improving, as well, their professional skills. A similar percentage (79%) indicate that the use of artificial intelligence is helpful in preventing burnout among healthcare workers. An effect that for medical staff means savings of up to 2/3 of reporting time, allowing 45% of physicians to spend more time talking to patients and performing surgeries or other procedures. But it doesn't end there, because artificial intelligence technologies allow us to make better predictions in treating diseases which has been shown to reduce the margin of error in treatment.

These are the main benefits found by a study conducted by innovative digital media company MIT - Technology Review Insights in collaboration with GE Healthcare, the medical division of General Electric that specializes in providing medical imaging equipment. More than 900 healthcare professionals (70 percent from the United States and the remaining 30 percent from the United Kingdom) participated in the study on the application of artificial intelligence in healthcare, including medical, business and management roles related to the procurement process or apply artificial intelligence, big data analytics or medical devices and technology.

Antonio Spera, CEO of GE Healthcare Italy, said artificial intelligence can not only increase the efficiency of processes, but also change the experience of healthcare professionals and their patients.In fact, the emerging trends are very encouraging, from clinical staff working with patients to the development of personalized treatments, and these are believed to be just the tip of the iceberg of the impact of smart technology on their lives.

Artificial intelligence must work for and with healthcare providers to create a robust and integrated ecosystem. The more humane the implementation of AI, the more it will be adopted and improve outcomes and return on investment.

According to the survey, the most interesting areas of use for artificial intelligence in healthcare are: optimization of patient flow management, where 65 percent of the sample is interested in implementing it and 39 percent have already adopted artificial intelligence technologies in this area, medical imaging and diagnostics (64 percent and 41 percent), automation of electronic medical records with natural language processing tools (63 percent and 43 percent), predictive analytics (63 percent and 40 percent) and patient data processing and risk analysis.

Indeed, AI can generate useful information to improve user efficiency, increase diagnostic accuracy, personalize care, improve the patient experience, and enable predictive and remote management of complex healthcare systems and tools.

4.4 The importance of the nurse's role in dementia education through technology

Technology can support care and improve the lives of people with dementia. Despite the large body of evidence demonstrating the benefits and opportunities offered by technology, there are still gaps in dementia care education regarding the consideration of technology and the ethics of it. It is critical to clarify that to maximize the ethical use of technology and improve outcomes, it must be incorporated into dementia education programs and widely available to the caregiving community.

Technology has the potential to transform dementia care. From traditional digital devices to dementia-specific systems, the technology continuum offers many opportunities for caregivers to develop their skills and be supported in their role. Examples of dementia-related technologies range from simple devices such as reminders, medication dispensers with reminders or GPS-tracking shoe parts to address the challenges of wandering, to more complex systems such as social robots designed to engage, calm and help frail individuals in everyday life. However, realizing the benefits of these tools requires a community of health technology professionals and the infrastructure to support it.

Traditional technologies such as tablets or online learning platforms can be used to effectively deliver dementia education to caregivers. Technology-based education uses interactive multimedia content to provide flexible learning opportunities that help caregivers determine what, when, and where learning takes place. It integrates with challenging care programs and has the potential to strengthen broad communities of caregivers in all locations. Virtual formats have become increasingly accessible, scalable, and affordable, and software developments such as augmented and virtual reality now offer new ways to enhance learning. Despite these opportunities, the use of technology in dementia education programs is not common. This is important because technology-based approaches can be used to significantly improve knowledge about dementia treatments.

Caregivers' opinions on the use of dementia methods vary. Many are curious and welcome the opportunity to discover how technology can support caregiving activities. According to a new study, 54 percent of caregivers would be less concerned about the safety of a person with dementia if they had the technology to support independent living. Others, however, fear that the devices require high technical skills to operate and therefore perceive the technology as stifling. Caregivers also expressed concern that the technology may have negative effects, including the potential to reduce caregivers' vigilance due to excessive technological activity. For caregivers over age 65, who make up 19 percent of the elderly population in the United States, barriers to dementia technology use may be exacerbated by low digital literacy, perceived distrust, and digital exclusion. Concerns about privacy, confidentiality, and autonomy create additional challenges for adoption, as both people with dementia and caregivers worry about unwanted disclosure of private or personally identifiable information. These challenges underscore the importance of strengthening caregivers' digital skills and equipping them with the tools to leverage existing solutions in a way that aligns with their values.

WHO's Global Action Plan to Combat Dementia Worldwide calls for international action to improve access to technological innovations that facilitate support for health care workers and improve their knowledge and skills. It has since been used throughout North America. The Dementia Strategy for Canada 'Together We Aspire' calls for increased readiness of health care providers to provide quality care through technology-based tools and resources. In the United States, the National Research Summit on Dementia Care and the National Alzheimer's Project Acts' Advisory Council on Alzheimer's Research, Care, and Services have identified dementia education and technology training as priority focus areas. The Alzheimer's Association Dementia Technology Professional Focus Area and the AGE-WELL NCE EPIC-AT programs are notable initiatives that have since been implemented in these countries to address these focus areas. Although such training programs help guide technology to optimize dementia care, they are largely limited to professional audiences; in fact, training offered to health care professionals is less developed.

To investigate public dementia education programs that might be readily available to general health care providers, some scholars relied on a Google search using the keywords 'dementia,' 'online,' 'education,' 'health care provider' and their synonyms. The top five pages of results contained 207 training programs from 89 service providers. Large differences were found in the quality and depth of training content and program characteristics such as delivery format, cost, duration, and state approval. Content analysis of course descriptions revealed that about 15% of program providers offered comprehensive training programs (scores $\geq$ 15 when coded with 20 dementia care topics, including nursing methods, communication, and wellness). Only 2% of providers mentioned this technology separately in their program descriptions. Programs rarely linked content to evidence-based sources, casting doubt on the credibility of teaching materials. Such scrutiny leaves room for the dissemination of false information or the use of predatory marketing tactics. These complexities make it difficult to identify and receive quality dementia education. Publicly available training on dementia treatments is particularly poor.

Technology continues to advance, and their use in dementia care is increasing. However, training programs that provide caregivers with the skills needed to use these technologies are still lagging behind.

It is necessary to close gaps in caregiver training and address the inequitable distribution of resources. It is well known that training healthy workers produces better outcomes. For caregivers, dementia training improves overall well-being and satisfaction with the role and significantly increases knowledge, attitude, and confidence. For supported clients, training leads to positive outcomes in terms of quality of life, communication, behavioral and psychological symptoms, and activities of daily living. It follows that empowering caregivers with skills to optimize technology for dementia can support autonomy, self-determination, and mutual benefit. Failure to provide caregivers with opportunities to strengthen their digital skills in dementia care technology can harm the people they are supposed to benefit. Equitable distribution of resources is important to protect the rights of people with dementia.

Information about technology needs to be transparent and openly evaluate promises against user concerns to build trust and break down barriers to adoption. Commonly cited concerns relate to the potential harms of data collection and digital surveillance from excessive surveillance and invasion of privacy. There are concerns about the storage and disclosure of personal or health-related information, particularly the potential unauthorized use of information by third-party companies or the sharing of sensitive information that leads to discrimination and stigmatization. Therefore, the responsible use of technology requires the provision of education and training to address these issues and increase awareness about the checks and balances that can be used to protect users' rights, providing people with the knowledge and skills to make informed decisions. The rapid development of the characteristics of dementia technologies and the growing importance of software such as artificial intelligence in healthcare environments further increase the urgency and centrality of education in the ethical adoption of technology. The promise of technology cannot translate into benefits if awareness remains low. Dementia treatments are at the crossroads of technology and medical ethics. Ethical, legal, and social issues related to the consequences of technology use overlap with the benefits and challenges of therapeutic practices. Protecting human rights and upholding these shared principles is therefore a task that should guide the development of dementia educational programming. The current educational environment is complex, sophisticated, and can be improved. With increasing pressure to increase care capacity, timely action is needed to fill gaps in caregiver training to enable people with dementia to ethically embrace technology and optimize it for living and thriving.

5. THE FUTURE OF DISEASE THROUGH TECHNOLOGICAL PROGRESS

5.1 Robotics: a model for Healthcare 4.0

In addition to the general development of work organization models, medicine is also moving toward the Healthcare 4.0 model. The model is characterized by human-centered healthcare services based on advanced digitization and automation of healthcare processes.

Its strength lies in implementing all emerging smart technologies: miniaturized sensors, wearables, advanced robotics, data storage systems, and anything that improves the effectiveness of care and promotes both prevention and active aging.

Robotics prevails in this scenario because it can be applied to healthcare systems aimed at surgery, diagnosis, rehabilitation, prosthetics, hospital logistics, and care for the elderly and disabled.

In general, the ideal target for robotic systems is all those procedures that require the performance of repetitive and well-structured tasks.

In particular, medical robotics consists of a series of high-tech applications that require the convergence of multidisciplinary skills such as mechanics, medicine, and computer science. This approach achieves a high level of patient care, simplifies clinical procedures, and creates a safe environment for patients and caregivers.

Medical applications are the most diverse, ranging from diagnosis to surgery, rehabilitation to neuroscience, monitoring of elderly and chronically ill patients, and intelligent and personalized treatments.

Robotic systems are increasingly finding applications in diagnostics, where they are supported by artificial intelligence aimed at digital interpretation of radiological and histopathological images.

With these methods it is possible to study parts of the human body that are difficult to reach with traditional instruments, which often cause discomfort for the patient.

In the field of rehabilitation, robotic devices can support or replace people. They are now rightly proposed for the following purposes:

-To meet the growing demand for human resources dedicated to rehabilitation;

-implement   more effective treatment protocols;

-reduces   medical staff fatigue.

Their use simplifies routine operations, ensures smoother processes, and offers patients more empathy and human interaction. The logistics side uses service robots that can monitor inventory, place timely orders and promote optimal placement of supplies, equipment and medicines.

In summary, it can be said that robotics will provide a concrete answer to the unprecedented increase in the health care needs of the aging population in the near future.

5.2 Robots for elderly care.

The assistive robot was developed by a consortium of experts from health care, the robotics industry, and dementia specialist groups.

The main feature of the robot is a user-oriented design method, with feedback in pilot studies coming from patients themselves.

The most interesting possibilities arise from the so-called Internet of Things, or the ability to connect devices and objects in the home and communicate with each other to improve the health, independence, and quality of life of the elderly or disabled.

Technology solutions specifically designed for the elderly can increase treatment adherence, perceived safety, and self-monitoring. In a study conducted by the Eurac Research Center in Bolzano, 36 South Tyroleans between the ages of 65 and 94 tested a home automation kit consisting of several Internet elements: a tablet, a clock with emergency mode, and sensors that were placed at strategic points in the home. This integrated system proved useful for monitoring the elderly's habits, monitoring their vital parameters, facilitating daily activities and alerting them to emergency situations. If, for example, a person habitually eats breakfast between seven and eight o'clock and does not open the refrigerator until nine o'clock, the sensor on the refrigerator sends a message to the tablet to make sure nothing has happened. If the person does not respond within 20 minutes, the system sends an alert to a loved one or caregiver so that someone can check on his or her condition. Other sensors control the automatic turning on of the light when the elderly person wakes up during the night, or the buzzer when the pot is left on the stove.

Another experiment at Nayang Technological University in Singapore showed that humanoid robots could be very useful in meeting the emotional and social needs of the elderly.

Pet robot Nadine-one of the most human-like features, interactions and behaviors in the world-entertained and entertained 29 residents over the age of 60 for several days at the Evergreen Nursing Home in Bright Hill, Singapore. Specifically, Nadine was tasked with running bingo games. All game sessions performed by the robot were filmed to compare the participants' reactions, facial expressions and behavior with those recorded when humans performed the same activity.

It turned out that the elderly felt more comfortable in the robot's company: their faces seemed more cheerful and smiling, their attention was higher and less distracted, and they avoided turning to the cane. Nadine's success depends mainly on her human-like appearance and ability to read gestures and facial expressions, key features that facilitate communication with the elderly, who are generally unaccustomed to technology.

A particularly effective health care strategy may be the development of technical systems that can compensate for the physical, cognitive, and behavioral deficits of people with dementia. The benefit, in addition to enabling the patient to become independent and continue to live at home, is to ease the physical and psychological burden on informal caregivers of caring for an increasingly common chronic, disabling and progressive disease. Assistive technologies that have proven to be effective in this area are again robots, particularly those responsible for rehabilitation, remote control, health assessment, and psychosocial support.

The most widely used semi-humanoid robot for this purpose is Pepper, which has been at IRCSS Casa Sollievo della Sofferenza in

San Giovanni Rotondo since October 2020 to help elderly people with cognitive decline and motor difficulties.

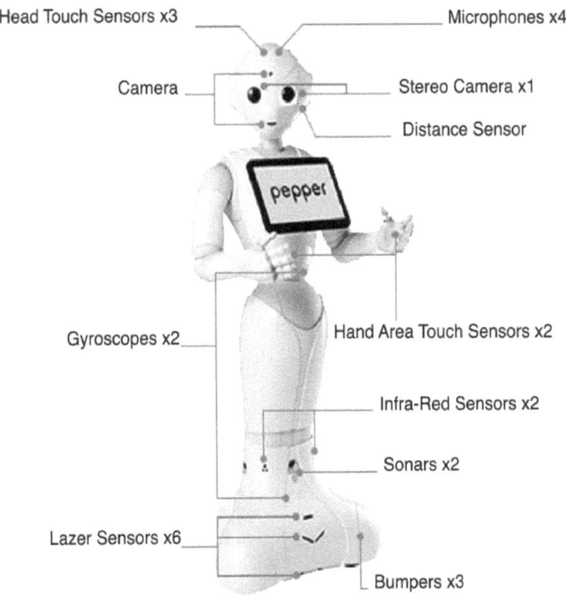

Studies show that paired clinical care interventions improve quality of life and social interaction and reduce the use of psychotropic and pain medications. In general, humanoid robots are mainly used for care and communication tasks, while robots with animal characteristics are used for emotional states.

All of these experiences open up suggestive scenarios for the versatile use of telemedicine, robotics, and home automation to improve the health of the elderly, combat social isolation, and slow cognitive decline.

However, these are experimental initiatives from which it is not yet possible to draw definitive and general conclusions. There is not enough information to assess the impact of robots and virtual assistants on the lives of the elderly, especially in the home environment. The quality of the studies conducted so far is also questioned, as it is difficult to directly involve people with dementia or disabilities in the design of machines according to user needs and expectations. In addition, ethical and legal difficulties remain regarding privacy protection, processing of personal data, and provision of informed consent, as well as practical problems due to the lack of digitization of citizens over 60 years of age.Although information technology allows for televised visits (remote medical consultations) and health monitoring with the help of portable medical devices, the hypothesis of delegating clinical and health tasks entirely to a robot or virtual assistant is not winning as a plausible alternative and is still much less desirable.

5.3 Artificial intelligence: the future serving the elderly

A study was recently conducted in Western countries, especially in Europe and the United States, on artificial intelligence in the care of the elderly and their approach. Both healthy individuals and individuals with typical disorders of the elderly (cognitive decline, frailty or depression) participated in various studies, which had as its main focus the work exercising AI in order to participate in the treatments and therapies of the elderly with dementia.

In a world where life expectancy is constantly increasing and where the average age of the population is rising at an alarming rate, an exponential increase in the prevalence of chronic diseases and high mortality in the population are inevitable. As a result, the care needs and desires of the elderly population are often not met because they exceed available resources, increasing the burden that health care systems around the world struggle to cope with. Therefore, it is important to find sustainable ways to promote the health of the elderly more effectively.

The rapid progress of AI-related projects, such as complex computer systems, can learn, solve problems, communicate with people through mechanisms that mimic human behavior, and perform various functions that can also be integrated into the healthcare setting.

An analysis of studies reveals that there is a wide range of artificial intelligence-based devices currently available in elderly care, and their roles may vary. For convenience, six categories of artificial intelligence have been identified: robots (humanoid and non-humanoid), exoskeletons, smart homes, wearable applications and devices, voice-activated devices, and virtual reality systems. These may in turn include five roles in as many domains: rehabilitation, emotional support, sociality, control, and thinking.

In rehabilitation A.I. has been used to restore motor function damaged by traumatic events, improve neglect, improve sleep quality, strengthen balance, prevent falls, and relieve pain.

As emotional support for elderly subjects, A.I. were able to improve their mood by reducing psychological stress, anxiety and depression. Regarding sociality, it has been found that AI. can promote contact between the elderly and their friends and family members, as well as strengthen relationships with caregivers. In addition, the integration of artificial intelligence through various services, such as streaming music or reading audiobooks, enables exposed individuals not only to be more cognitively active, but also to participate more socially because they have more conversational cues.

It allows the elderly person to be monitored at different levels and helps both the person, for example, the time of taking the medication, and the health care providers caring for the elderly person, for example, by collecting a number of useful parameters to choose the one best suited for his or her clinical course.

In the role of cognitive initiator, A.I. knows how to support the elderly with the goal of slowing their cognitive decline or alleviating cognitive-behavioral symptoms in people who have already been diagnosed with cognitive impairment.

It is also necessary to consider that several studies have pointed to the need to find new ways to help the elderly in a more comprehensive way that also meets the needs of health care providers, because they often tend to become stressed due to the inability to recover and sometimes the inability to recognize symptoms and needs due to the lack of adequate health care culture. The overall impact of artificial intelligence-based technologies and approaches to elderly care seems promising, especially considering that various artificial intelligence systems have generally been able to meet health and personal needs that are often overlooked in the elderly and infirm.

It is clear that AI-based devices must be provided in an age-appropriate manner to overcome barriers related to distrust in the benefits of new technologies.

Studies conducted show that not only the number of available technologies is increasing, but also their diversity, allowing them to be increasingly integrated into the health sector.

Technologies currently based on A.I. combine machine learning techniques with increasingly sophisticated computer algorithms to meet increasingly complex needs, including business and entertainment needs, facilitating communication and enhancing social interaction. In addition, the devices are designed to be even safer, easier, and more fun to make them even more accessible to older people.

All this promotes the elderly person's autonomy, enables him to profitably carry out his daily activities, and offers psychosocial support.

Most artificial intelligence-based healthcare devices have yet to be implemented in clinical practice, so healthcare professionals and institutions may be reluctant to offer these technologies to real recipients in the absence of clinical validation. Future research should therefore focus on clinical validation of AI-based devices and their increasing prevalence in the profession to bridge the gap between theory and practice.

5.4 The Italian state's investment in advanced technology

The Italian government wants to support new startup investments in artificial intelligence.

On Artificial Intelligence Day, they talked about the opportunities and risks of artificial intelligence, the need for its careful regulation and monitoring, but also, and most importantly, supporting local talent by turning ideas into something concrete.

In his end-of-year message 2023, President Sergio Mattarella reminded how important it is to be able to read the direction and speed of the changes we are experiencing. Changes that can have a positive impact on our lives. Technology has always changed economic and social structures. Now it is producing unstoppable development with the help of self-sustaining artificial intelligence, thought to profoundly change our professional, social and interpersonal habits. The President of the Republic reminds us that we are in the midst of what is remembered as a great historical leap at the beginning of the third millennium, so it must be ensured that the current revolution remains human. It is written in the tradition of a civilization that sees man - and his dignity - as a necessary pillar of support.

The current government has decided to revise the strategic plan for the three-year period 2022-2024 drawn up by the Draghi government in 2021 before its natural expiration. This is an entirely acceptable choice, also because the plan that came about thanks to good work had several limitations, as these columns already pointed out at the time. Apart from a too short time and space horizon (three years and main focus on research and development), it had no special budget or management. Two deadly sins that we believe the developing strategy will solve, because to be really sharp and no longer a new dreambook, the strategy needs to show, on the one hand, realistically available figures and, on the other hand, the actors responsible for the planned activities and the mechanism for monitoring their implementation and its effects .

So far, there are mainly two government initiatives that are expected to find a place in the strategy, according to public rumors. The most macroscopic one in terms of size is undoubtedly the creation of a public-private investment fund under the aegis of CDP to foster the growth of Italian innovative startups.

In fact, when considering venture capital investments in artificial intelligence, Italy is outperformed not only by France and Germany (often by multiples) and Spain, but also by much smaller countries such as the Netherlands and Sweden. A fund certainly cannot work miracles, but if managed properly and especially in combination with existing funds and with funds that may be attractive from abroad (think of some recent activity in Europe, especially in France and Germany, where the key players are in the U.S. capital) it could significantly accelerate the current growth trajectory.

In this context, where Italy has smaller and often very small businesses compared to other countries, the tax incentives for digital education (so-called "education 4.0") planned until 2022 appear particularly relevant. But the overall review of business incentives from the transition from 4.0 to 5.0 is an important test case. After so many announcements for 2023, the new arrangement should finally see the light of day early in the new year, after lengthy negotiations with the European Commission on the recently approved amendment to the NRP.

The danger just mentioned is that when green transition and energy efficiency are included in the underdeveloped 4.0 paradigm, neither transition, and especially the country's competitiveness, which should be the main benefit of support measures. In a technological climate of great change, entrepreneurs, especially smaller ones, should be supported not only and perhaps not primarily by financial incentives to purchase hardware or software, but also by expertise that does not need to know the investments best suited to the situation.

This gives rise to measures such as coupons to purchase innovative consulting services from accredited entities of the 4.0 (or 5.0) overhaul, which consist of comparing the state of the technologies used with the best competitors in the industry. in the field and a specific plan to scale the technology level. In such a framework, financial incentives would complement that process of efficient growth tailored to real business needs (including through artificial intelligence), avoiding unprofitable government and/or corporate investment.

The year 2024 will finally be the year when such a cultural leap in innovative policy can be made, although there are still many doubts due in part to the many external and internal limitations of the state budget and the ability of the public administration to think in these terms, but hope must never be given up.

CONCLUSION

After taking a comprehensive view of Alzheimer's disease, the conclusion was reached to test new treatments and use technology in order to prevent it and diagnose it early.

From the analysis of numerous research studies, new ways of experimentation have emerged such as the use of new artificial neural networks and the first artificial neuron on a microchip that will help solve some problems related to the field of medicine, but most importantly will help those who are mainly affected by Alzheimer's disease.

Through the implementation of research with artificial intelligence, the nurse and other healthcare professionals will need to acquire continuing education such that a new approach based on advanced technology will be provided to the patient.

With the use of artificial intelligence, it has been possible to develop a new model of care that involves the use of humanoid robots capable of improving the health and independence of the elderly, although it should be made clear that they can never completely replace the emotions of caregivers.

However, the future study of Alzheimer's disease is expected to be centered through the use of technology, so the Health System will contribute in the investment by moving from a 4.0 to a 5.0 model of digital education by improving research for the study of neurodegenerative diseases.

BIBLIOGRAPHY

1. A History of Neuropsychology (Frontiers of Neurology and Neuroscience Book 44) 1st Edition, by J. Bogousslavsky (Editor), F. Boller (Editor), M. Iwata (Editor) Format: Kindle Edition. Part of: Frontiers of Neurology and Neuroscience (17 books).

2. Territo Dana, Alzheimer's Q&A: What are the five 'A's' of Alzheimer's disease?, "The Advocate," Feb 16 2020

3. Baldereschi M, Di Carlo A, Maggi s, Inzitari D (2002). Dementias: epidemiology and risk factors. In Le Demenze, 3rd edition, Marco Trabucchi, UTET.

4. Costanza Papagno, Nadia Bolognini: Neuropsychology of dementias, Il Mulino (2020). Series: Aspects of Psychology.

5. Stefano Govoni, Federica Del Signore, Alessia Rosi, Stefano F. Cappa, Nicola Allegri, 'Dementias: pharmacological and nonpharmacological treatment and caregiver stress management', Journal Italian Society of General Medicine no. 5 - vol. 27 - 2020.

6. Cummings J, Lee G, Ritter A, et al. Alzheimer's disease drug development pipeline: 2020. Alzheimer's & Dementia: Translational Research & Clinical Interventions 2020;6:e12050

7. Guaita A, Trabucchi M. Dementias. Care and treatment. Maggioli Editore 2016.

8. Takeda M, Tanaka T, Okochi M, et al. Nonpharmacological intervention for dementia patients. Psychiatry Clin Neurosci 2012.

9. Griffin, J. M., Riffin, C., Havyer, R. D., Biggar, V. S., Comer, M., Frangiosa, T. L., & Bangerter, L. R. (2019). Integrating Family Caregivers of People With Alzheimer's Disease and Dementias into Clinical Appointments: Identifying Potential Best Practices. Journal of Applied Gerontology.

10. Nolan, L. (2006). Caring connections with older persons with dementia in an acute hospital setting ? a hermeneutic interpretation of the staff nurse's experience. International Journal of Older People Nursing.

11. Arenaza-Urquijo EM, Vemuri P. Resistance vs resilience to Alzheimer disease: clarifying terminology for preclinical studies. Neurology 2018

12. Stern Y, Arenaza-Urquijo EM, Bartrés-Faz D, et al. Whitepaper: defining and investigating cognitive reserve, brain reserve and brain maintenance. Alzheimers Dement 2018

13. Wu L, Sun D. Adherence to Mediterranean diet and risk of developing cognitive disorders: an updated systematic review and meta-analysis of prospective cohort studies. Sci Rep 2017

14. Dafsari FS, Jessen F. Depression - an underrecognized target for prevention of dementia in Alzheimer's disease. Translational Psychiatry 2020

15. Manickam P, Mariappan SA, Murugesan SM, Hansda S, Kaushik A, Shinde R, Thipperudraswamy SP. Artificial Intelligence (AI) and Internet of Medical Things (IoMT) Assisted Biomedical Systems for Intelligent Healthcare. Biosensors (Basel). 2022 Jul 25;12(8):562. doi: 10.3390/bios12080562. PMID: 35892459; PMCID: PMC9330886

16. Martin, Susanna E., Tam, Mallorie T., and Robillard, Julie M.. 'Technology in Dementia Education: An Ethical Imperative in a Digitized World'. 1 Jan. 2024

17. Ablameyko S., Goras L., Gori M., Piuri V.: Limitations and Future Trends in Neural Computation. IOS Publishing, (Eds 2003).

18. Angluin D., Smith C.: Inductive inference: theory and methods. Computing Surveys, Vol. 15, No. 3, 1983

19. Dosso JA , Bandari E , Malhotra A , Hoey J , Michaud F , Prescott TJ , Robillard JM ((2022)) Towards emotionally aligned social robots for dementia: Perspectives of care partners and persons with dementia. Alzheimers Dement 18: , e059261.

20. Ienca M , Wangmo T , Jotterand F , Kressig RW , Elger B ((2018)) Ethical design of intelligent assistive technologies for dementia: A descriptive review. Sci Eng Ethics 24

21. Ryan AA , McCauley CO , Laird EA , Gibson A , Mulvenna MD , Bond R , Bunting B , Curran K , Ferry F ((2020)) 'There is still so much inside': The impact of personalized reminiscence, facilitated by a tablet device,

on people living with mild to moderate dementia and their family carers. Dementia 19

22. Robillard JM , Wu JM , Feng TL , Tam MT ((2019)) Prioritizing benefits: A content analysis of the ethics in dementia technology policies. J Alzheimers Dis 69

23. Wójcik D , Szczechowiak K , Konopka P , Owczarek M , Kuzia A , Rydlewska-Liszkowska I , Pikala M ((2021)) Informal dementia caregivers: Current technology use and acceptance of technology in care. Int J Environ Res Public Health 18

24. Knapp M , Barlow J , Comas-Herrera A , Damant J , Freddolino P , Hamblin K , Hu B , Lorenz K , Perkins M , Rehill A , Wittenberg R , Woolham J (2015) The case for investment in technology to manage the global costs of dementia, Policy Innovation Research Unit, London, United Kingdom.

25. Marston HR , Musselwhite CBA ((2021)) Improving older people's lives through digital technology and practices. Gerontol Geriatr Med 7

26. Alzheimer's Disease International (2022) World Alzheimer's Report 2022. Life after diagnosis: Navigating treatment, care and support. Alzheimer's Disease International, London, England.

27. Jones C , Jones D , Moro C ((2021)) Use of virtual and augmented reality-based interventions in health education to improve dementia knowledge and attitudes: An integrative review. BMJ Open 11

28. Newbould L , Samsi K , Wilberforce M ((2022)) Developing effective workforce training to support the long-term care of older adults: A review of reviews. Health Soc Care Community 30

29. Berridge C , Turner NR , Liu L , Fredriksen-Goldsen KI , Lyons KS , Demiris G , Kaye J , Lober WB ((2023)) Preliminary efficacy of let's talk tech: Technology use planning for dementia care dyads. Innov Aging 7

30. Kristiansen S , Beck M , Kabir ZN , Konradsen H ((2022)) Providing dementia care using technological solutions: An exploration of caregivers' and dementia coordinators' experiences. J Clin Nurs

31. Hicks B , Karim A , Jones E , Burgin M , Cutler C , Tang W , Thomas S , Nyman SR ((2022)) Care home practitioners' perceptions of the barriers and facilitators for using off-the-shelf gaming technology with people with dementia. Dementia 21

32. Felber NA , Tian (Angelina) YJ , Pageau F , Elger BS , Wangmo T ((2023)) Mapping ethical issues in the use of smart home health technologies to care for older persons: A systematic review. BMC Med Ethics 24

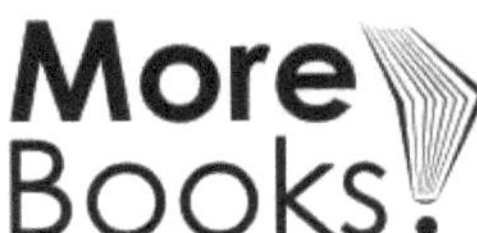

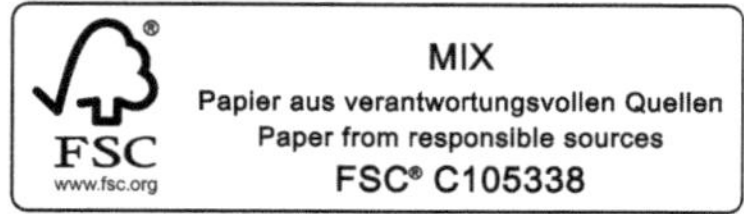

Printed by Books on Demand GmbH, Norderstedt / Germany